DAR LEMMON

Guide To Essential Oils

Natural Healing for everyday aches and pains, including recipes.

This book was professionally typeset on Reedsy.
Find out more at reedsy.com

Contents

1

Introduction

Introduction

Hello my name is Darlene Lemmon. I am excited to write this quick guide to essential oils for everyday aches and pains.

I got into essential oils a few years back. I had bad allergies due to ragweed blooming in the fall. It was so bad I was talking about six allergy relief pills a day just to cope. I knew that couldn't be good for me. So I started looking for other options to ease my discomfort after going to the doctor and all they wanted to do was pop more harsh drugs in me as well.

A nephew of mine and his wife are big into natural healing and they told me of an app that they used to learn about essential oils and their usages. I'll list this in the resources for you. But that had really opened my eyes about natural healing instead of using modern medicine. I started doing a lot more research and finding things that not only helped my allergies but also headache, joint inflammation and so many other pains that we get just from our bodies aging.

I see so many people that suffer from medical conditions that natural healing would help and be easier on their bodies than taking over the counter medicines. I'm hoping this book will help people like that and be cheaper on their pocket books also.

I thought a book with some of the recipes that I use for normal aches and pains would be a great resource for others. I normally write my recipes down in a notebook. Having a physical copy about the basics of essential oils with recipes I thought would be better . You can jot down anything you may add or take away to make these recipes, change them up to your own liking.

I will definitely buy one of these books for myself and family members to have at their fingertips when they need it. Be like having a good cookbook with all your favorite meals in it for easy access.

Hope you enjoy the book.

2

History of Essential Oils

History of Essential Oils

When I started looking into essential oils, I did some digging into the ancient days before modern medicine ever came about. How did people heal themselves of their aches and pains back in the old days? I won't go too deep into the history, just a little bit of background on essential oils.

Back in the ancient Egyptian days somewhere around 4500 BC essential oils were used more for cosmetic and ointmental reasons. They would even mix up herbal solutions before burying the dead. Think that was their way of embalming a body before burial.

It was Chinese and Indian that started using essential oils more for medicine in around 3000 to 2000 BC. They had a much bigger list of essential oils that they used than the ancient Egyptians did. China and India used around 600 to 700 different oils for healing purposes.

Then the Greeks finally jumped on the essential oil wagon around 500 to 400 BC. They added even more essential oils to the list as well that had not yet been discovered earlier.

Just a few years ago around the 19th century some of the active ingredients in the medical plants started getting recorded. The chemist started realizing the importance of some of the active ingredients that could help with relieving pain and help heal people of certain ailments.

Fast forward to today's time. More and more people like you and I are realizing the same thing; that there really are healing properties in essential oils.

The wise tails and old remedies that our ancestors tried to teach us are true.

3

Understanding of Essential Oils

Understanding of Essential Oils

Essential oils are made from pretty much the whole plant. They use the flower, leaves, bark, stem, roots, every part of the plant or tree to extract the oil from it. It is cold pressed to make the oil.

Some oils can be pretty strong and people react differently to them. Essential oils can be used in a few different ways. Depending on what aches and pains you are trying to treat. You can use it by aromatic diluting the oil in water in a diffuser. Topical mixing in a carrier oil or to make lotion to put directly on your skin. Or inhaling the essential oils like for sinus issues I would put a drop or two of eucalyptus in the palm of my hand, cup my nose with palms and inhale.

It is always good to mix the oils with what they call a carrier oil. Carrier oils are just oils to dilute the essential oils in, so they aren't so strong. Some people may have allergic reactions from them. It's always good to test them out with just a drop or two in your carrier oil not to make it too strong till you know you're good with it.

4

Essential Oils VS Modern Medicine

Essential Oils VS Modern Medicine

Essential oils are naturally made from the plants and trees. They are safe to use if used properly. Diluting them is the safest way to use them. Be cautious when using on small children, they are more sensitive to these oils than adults are.

When it comes to modern medicine. They normally cost more than the essential oils do. Considering that it only takes a few drops in some carrier oil to make your healing lotion. The bottle of essential oil can go a long way.

Modern medicine has chemicals in it that most of us can't even pronounce. Some of the medicine has several ingredients that are damaging to our organs if taken for a long time. This in the long run can do more damage than good.

Safety using oils with certain health conditions

If you are on any kind of modern medicine, please check with your doctor to make sure the essential oils you are wanting to try don't affect your medicine. I have heard that some oils will counteract with certain medicines. For example grapefruit essentials may counteract with high blood pressure medicine. Just be very cautious if you are on medicine of any kind to call and get your doctor's advice before using certain essential oils.

5

Best Essential Oils for Everyday Aches and Pains

Best Oils for Everyday Aches and Pains

Here is a list of essential oils and their properties and uses. This is a list of essential oils I use the most for everyday aches and pains. I didn't list all of their properties and usages, just the ones that I thought are most known to people. I did list uses that are more serious too. I know so many people out there that suffer from more serious illnesses like cancer, high blood pressure, cataracts, kidney stones, etc. I hope this will help those of you reading this that may suffer from more serious pains not just the normal aches. I gave a brief description of what I use each one for. I know several of them have a lot of the same properties. Some work better than others for different ailments.

- **Lavender**

Properties

Anticoagulant, anticonvulsant, antidepressant, antifungal, antihistamine, anti-infectious, anti-inflammatory, antiseptic.

<u>Uses</u>
Acne, Allergies, Anxiety, Blisters, Bug repellent, Burns, Calming, Depression, Diaper rash, Dry skin, High Blood Pressure, Inflammation, Sleep, Stress, Tension, Wrinkles and so much more.

Lavender is one of my most go to essential oils. I use it for so many things. It is great to put a few drops in a diffuser and make the house smell good. As it is refreshing the air it is also helping me relax before bedtime.

I use lavender also for cleaning the floors. I mix it with 50/50 water and vinegar, it helps kill the vinegar smell.

• Eucalyptus

<u>Properties</u>
Antibacterial, anti-infectious, anti-inflammatory, antiseptic, antiviral, diuretic, insect repellent, and stimulant.

<u>Uses</u>
Asthma, bronchitis, carpal tunnel, cataracts, congestion, coughs, deodorant, emphysema, fever, high blood pressure, hypoglycemia, inflammation, kidney stones, migraine headaches, pain, sinusitis, sore throat, strep throat and more.

Eucalyptus is my go to essential oil for sinus issues. When I'm congested due to allergies it works great. Just a drop behind the ears clears my sinus or if real congested I will put a drop or two in the palm of my hand and inhale it through my nose.

Eucalyptus is really good in a diffuser at night time as well. This will help clear your sinuses while you sleep.

• Peppermint

<u>Properties</u>

Analgesic, antibacterial, anticarcinogenic, anti-inflammatory (prostate and nerves), antiseptic, antiviral and invigorating.

<u>Uses</u>

Alertness, allergies, antibacterial, antioxidants, asthma, autism, bad breath, carpal tunnel, chronic fatigue, cold sores, concentration, cramps, diarrhea, fever, flu, headaches, heartburn, hot flashes, muscle fatigue, nausea and so much more.

Peppermint is really good for allergies also but I use it more for headaches. If you put a couple drops on your temples and/or on your neck close to the base of the skull it could help ease the pain.

Peppermint is also good in a diffuser to help relieve allergies and make the house smell good.

• Tea Tree

<u>Properties</u>

Antibacterial, antifungal, anti-infectious, anti-inflammatory, antioxidant, antiparasitic, strong antiseptic, antiviral, digestive, insecticidal to name a few.

<u>Uses</u>

Acne, allergies, athlete's foot, cavities, cold sores, colds, coughs, dandruff, deodorant, earache, flu, gum disease, infection (skin), inflammation, rashes, sore throat, strep throat and wounds.

I like tea tree essential oil when I get cold sores. It takes the pain and infection away so fast. Still takes a few days for the cold sore to go away completely but the tea tree keeps the pain and discomfort away.

I also have used tea tree oil when I made homemade deodorant and toothpaste. I have good dentist visits every time so I really think it works good for cavities and gum disease.

• Frankincense

Properties

Anticancer, antidepressant, anti-infectious, anti-inflammatory, antiseptic, antitumoral and immune-stimulant.

Uses

Arthritis, asthma, concussion, confusion, coughs, depression, infection (skin), inflammation, mental fatigue, tumors, ulcer, warts, wrinkles and much more.

Frankincense is great for making lotions for arthritis. I have also made a homemade mouthwash rinse with a couple drops of frankincense in it.

• Clary Sage

Properties

Anticonvulsive, antifungal, antiseptic, antispasmodic, astringent, nerve tonic, soothing, tonic and warming.

Uses

Autism, cholesterol, cramps (abdominal), Epilepsy, hair loss, hot flashes, seizure.

After someone in the house has been sick I would put clary sage in a diffuser to help kill any germs that may be in the air.

- **Oregano**

Properties
Antibacterial, antifungal, antiparasitic, antiseptic, antiviral.
Uses
Calluses, parasites, pneumonia, sore throat and viral infection.

Oregano is a very strong essential oil, always dilute it with carrier oil. I use it more for DIY cleaning disinfectant spray. It is great at killing germs, mixed with other essential oils along with water and apple cider vinegar for a cleaning agent.

- **Lemon**

Properties
Antiseptic, antifungal, antioxidant, antiviral and refreshing.
Uses
Air purification, antioxidant, anxiety, bathroom and kitchen cleaning, carpets, colds, constipation, dishes, disinfectant, fever, furniture polish, laundry, overeating, relaxation, stress and water purification.

Lemon is my go to essential oil for an all purpose cleaner for my bathroom and kitchen. It is great for disinfecting counters, tubs and toilets, and also leaves a nice clean refreshing smell.

• Grapefruit

<u>Properties</u>

Antidepressant, antiseptic, disinfectant, stimulant, and tonic.

<u>Uses</u>

Appetite suppressant, hangovers, indigestion, obesity, overeating, and weight loss.

For indigestion I would rather eat the fruit than to make a tonic from the essential oil. The oil is good to put in a diffuser to help stimulate you in the mornings or give you a boost of energy before a workout.

• Lemongrass

<u>Properties</u>

Analgesic, antibacterial, anticancer, anti-inflammatory, antiseptic, insect repellent, and more.

<u>Uses</u>

Air purification, carpal tunnel, cataracts, cholesterol, varicose veins and more.

Lemongrass is good to make DIY insect repellents. It is also good to clean the air and put in a diffuser as an air purifier. It is supposed to help with vision if put around your eye. Caution not to get it too close to your eyes. I tried that once even putting it way around my eye it burned pretty bad. I didn't do that again, ha ha.

• Rosemary

Properties

Antibacterial, anticancer, antifungal, anti-infectious, anti-inflammatory, antioxidant, and expectorant.

Uses

Alcoholism, arthritis, autism, colds, constipation, diabetes, flu, hair loss, headaches, memory, mental support, muscle cramps, and much more.

I have used rosemary lotion for my hands, my arthritis has not bothered me since. I really like it for that reason.

- **Thyme**

Properties

Highly antibacterial, antifungal, antioxidant, antiviral, and antiseptic.

Uses

Aging, bronchitis, colds, eczema, sciatica, spider bites, viral infection and more.

I never think of thyme as a healing herb. I use it for cooking every now and then but that's about it. I will definitely have to try to make lotion with it. I have a great nephew with eczema and I get sciatica every once in a while. I will have to test thyme out and see if it works.

- **Geranium**

Properties

Antibacterial, antidepressant, antioxidant, antiseptic, insect repellent, refreshing, relaxing, and sedative.

Uses
Air purification, autism, bleeding, bruises, chapped lips, diarrhea, dry skin, physical stress, and sensitive skin.

I really like using geranium essential oil in my wash. When I wash my bedding or the dogs and cats bedding it smells so good afterwards. It is very pleasant to lay down on fresh clean sheets that smell like geranium. I have other flowery essential oils that I use for the laundry as well. Like rose, violet, lilac, gardenia and freesia.

- **German Chamomile**

Properties
Analgesic, antifungal, anti-infectious, anti-inflammatory, antioxidant, digestive tonic.
Uses
Acne, chapped lips, eczema, teething pain, and ulcer.

I've used German chamomile in homemade lotions and in homemade chapstick. I don't have eczema but it really helped in the winter months with the dry weather.

- **Helichrysum**

Properties
Antibacterial, anticoagulant, antioxidant, anticatarrhal, and antiviral.
Uses
Bleeding, blood clots, bone (bruised), bruises, burns, cholesterol, eczema, nose bleed, scarring, sciatica, sun screen, tinnitus, and more.

Helichrysum, it's a bit tough trying to pronounce that one. This essential oil is good for lotions and making facial creams. Helichrysum is good for anti-aging and rejuvenating damaged skin.

More study has come out that it is supposed to be good for weight loss as well.

6

Carrier Oils

C**arrier Oils to be used with Essential Oils**

Carrier oils are very important to blend your essential oils with. Some essential oils are too strong to be used as is without diluting it first in a carrier oil. Carrier oils help them soak into your skin better and not evaporate too quickly.

Carrier oils also have some healing properties as well which could boost the healing process.

- **Coconut oil**

Coconut oil has a lot of health benefits as well which makes it a really good carrier oil to use with essential oils. It promotes stress relief, strengthens hair, can improve dental health, absorbs great into the skin, helps with blood sugar levels, can boost metabolism, improve blood pressure and cholesterol as well. It has so many health benefits just by itself which makes it a great carrier oil to use with essential oils.

• Sweet Almond oil

Sweet almond oil is great for homemade lotions and facial creams. This oil absorbs fast into the skin and helps hydrate dry skin. Sweet almond oil has anti-inflammatory and emollient properties which makes it a great oil to use on damaged skin and can help with complexion and toning your skin.

• Jojoba Oil

Jojoba oil is an all around good oil to use. It not only moisturizes your dry skin but can help heal small sores, and reduce wrinkles. Jojoba oil has antioxidant properties like vitamin A and E along with omega 6 which will help your overall skin condition.

• Grapeseed oil

Grapeseed oil has a plethora of benefits which makes it a fantastic carrier oil to use. It could help lower your bad cholesterol (LDL) which would assist in lowering blood pressure. Improve your blood circulation and lower the risk of blood clots. Reduce inflammation, inflammation is linked to so many diseases and illnesses anything you can do to help that would improve your health dramatically.

Grapeseed oil can be used when making tonics for allergies to fight histamines that cause a lot of allergy symptoms. Could also make a homemade neosporin to use to help heal cuts and scrapes.

- **Plum Oil**

Is really good for making lotions, hair and nail homemade treatments. Plum carrier oil has anti-inflammatory properties, it quickly soaks in to hydrate your skin. Another reason this is a good carrier oil is that it is noncomedogenic so it won't clog your pores. Can be used to clean the face, remove makeup and be good for making lotion for dry skin and eczema.

- **Rosehip Oil**

Rosehip has fatty acids and antioxidants that help retain water and helps repair damaged skin. Is a lot like plum carrier oil, for the fact that it is another noncomedogenic oil that won't clog the pores in the skin. Rosehip will be great to use in lotions and facial creams, hair and nail treatments as well.

- **Olive Oil**

Olive oil isn't just for cooking anymore. It can be used as a carrier oil also.

Make sure you get a good quality Extra Virgin Olive oil. This oil is high in good fatty acids which is why it is used for cooking. This is why it can be used also as a carrier oil, it will help moisturize your skin and cleanse your face. This oil works great for making homemade soaps as well.

- **Argan Oil**

Argan oil is another carrier oil that is good to be used in lotions and massage oils. Its properties consist of Vitamins A and E as well as having monounsaturated fatty acids. It is an anti-inflammatory oil good for rejuvenating damaged dry skin. Argan oil will help with eczema, damaged hair and possibly reduce wrinkles.

- **Avocado Oil**

I just love avocado oil when it comes to cooking and making homemade salad dressings. But it can also be great as a carrier oil when making body lotions. Avocado oil has oleic acid and monounsaturated fatty acids making it great for dry skin.

- **Sunflower Oil**

Is another cooking oil that can be used as a carrier oil. It is known to protect skin from toxins and germs. Use this oil for massage oils or in body lotion recipes.

- **Black Seed Oil**

Black seed oil properties consist of saturated and unsaturated fatty acids along with possible anti-inflammatory properties. This makes it good for an all around skin care oil to use for eczema and acne.

I listed more carrier oils than I actually use. This will give you a wide variety to choose from and there are more out there also that I didn't name.

I didn't go into the history of how each is made. Figured you can always look that information up if you are interested.

Keep in mind that some of these oils are heavier than others. When making facial creams or cleansers use the lighter oils that won't clog your pores and cause acne.

7

Essential Oil Recipes

Recipes

Migraine Headaches

- ¼ c liquid coconut oil or any other carrier oil of your choice, like jojoba oil, grapeseed oil, sweet almond oil
- 4 drops peppermint oil
- 2 drop lavender oil

Mix all three in a dark bottle. Then pour into a roller bottle or just use a finger tip to massage into your temples. Rub some on the back of neck at the base of skull as well.

Tension Headaches

- 1 tsp coconut oil or any other carrier oil of your choice, like jojoba oil, grapeseed oil, sweet almond oil
- 2 drop peppermint oil

Mix together in a dark bottle and rub on the back of the neck at the base of the skull.

Eczema Lotion

- 1/2 c coconut oil,any other carrier oil of your choice
- 12 drops lavender
- 12 drops German chamomile

Mix all together and massage into eczema spots.

Arthritis

- 1/2 c coconut oil, any other carrier oil of your choice, like jojoba oil, grapeseed oil, sweet almond oil
- 12 drops Rosemary
- 12 drops Frankincense

Mix well in a glass jar and massage into joints were needed.

Anxiety

- 2 drops lavender
- 2 drops eucalyptus
- 2 drops frankincense

Put in a diffuser to help calm you down if at home. Can mix these three with 3 to 4 tsp of a carrier oil to take on the go.
Or

- 2 drops lavender

- 2 drops German chamomile
- 3 tsp coconut oil, any other carrier oil of your choice, like jojoba oil, grapeseed oil, sweet almond oil

Mix all together in a dark bottle or roller bottle. Massage on wrist, behind ears, back of neck for absorption and to help you relax.

Insomnia

- 5 drops lavender

Or

- 5 drops geranium

Place into a diffuser to help relax you to fall asleep. Both of these are really good to help relax after a busy day.

Flu and Colds

- 5 drops tea tree
- 2 drops thyme
- 2 drops rosemary
- 2 drops frankincense

Mix in a diffuser to help fight cold and flu while you rest. There are so many ways to mix and match essential oils to fight off colds, flus and coughs. Can add eucalyptus, clove, lemon and other essential oils that have antiviral, anti-infectious and anti-inflammatory properties.

Congestion

- 1 tsp coconut oil or oil of your choice
- 2 drops peppermint

Mix well and rub on the chest to help relieve congestion.

Inflammation Joints

- ½ c coconut oil, any other carrier oil of your choice, like jojoba oil, grapeseed oil, sweet almond oil
- 8 drops lavender
- 8 drops frankincense
- 8 drops tea tree

Mix well in a dark bottle then rub into aching joints. Recipes for inflammatory joints work well for arthritis also.

Toothaches

- 1 tsp coconut oil
- 2 drops of clove oil

Mix together and rub around the tooth that hurts. Coconut oil is great for dental health. Can also just suck on a whole clove, sometimes this works better than trying to get the oil on the tooth.

Muscle aches

- 1/2 c coconut oil, any other carrier oil of your choice, like jojoba oil, grapeseed oil, sweet almond oil
- 6 drops lavender
- 6 drops frankincense

- 6 drops lemongrass
- 6 drops tea tree

Mix well in a dark bottle then massage into strained muscle. There's several different essential oils you can use for sore muscles. Mix and match whichever ones you prefer.

Cuts and Scrapes

- 1 tsp coconut oil or other type of carrier oil
- 2 drops lavender
- 1 drop tea tree oil

Mix well and dab onto the wound for fast healing and keep from getting infected.

Insect Bites

- ¼ c coconut oil
- 6 drops lavender
- 3 drops Tea tree
- 3 drops peppermint

Mix well then rub onto the insect bite. Use liquid coconut oil or any other liquid carrier oil to use in a roller bottle.

8

Measuring Ratios And Equipment

Measuring Ratio: Carrier Oil to Drops of Essential Oils

As a rule of thumb to mix essential oils with carrier oils, it is good to remember the ratio mixture is 1 teaspoon carrier oil to 2 drops of essential oils. So the way I calculated the number of drops of essential oils to the carrier oils is:

- 48 teaspoons equals 1 cup
- 24 teaspoons equals ½ cup
- 12 teaspoons equals ¼ cup

Depending on how large of a batch you are making, whether using a cup, 1/2 c, ¼ c or just a few teaspoons. You would take the essential oils you are wanting to use in your recipe and decide how many drops of each oil you want to use to equal that many drops per ratio of the carrier oil. You can do equal drops of each oil or more drops of one than the other. There are endless ways of mixing and matching the essential oils to come up with a recipe that you like and that works well for you.

Equipment

The dark bottles, spray bottles and roller bottles can be bought online at several different online stores. There are small, like very small funnels that can be bought as well to help when pouring the carrier oils into the small bottles. They really help and keep from making such a mess when making recipes.

There are also small tools that can be purchased to help take the little plastic dropper pieces in and out of the essential oil bottles and remove and install the rollers that go into the roller bottles.

These little accessory tools will make things so much easier when making recipes.

9

Conclusion

C onclusion

I hope you have enjoyed this book. These recipes are more of a basic starter point to get you going if you are new to essential oils. I didn't want to go too much into the history of each essential oils on how they are made. Thought that would be too much to get into as beginners to essential oils.

If you notice I used coconut oil a lot as my carrier oil. It has so many great health benefits that accompany a lot of the essential oils. By all means use whichever carrier oil you like, definitely try the others as well. Depending on what recipe your making will help determine which carrier oil to use. There are more carrier oils out there to choose from. I just listed the ones that are more well known and used more often.

There are tons of essential oils out there more than I can count. The ones I listed are more of the common ones. A lot of the essential oils have similar if not the same property and uses. Some I feel work better than others. But they all have different smells, there are some I just don't care for because of their smell. Try different formulas and different essential oils to see which ones you like. You will always find one that you like that will help with your aches and pains.

There are a few apps out there that you can upload on your phone that will help tremendously. The one I use is the Reference Guide for Essential Oils, it is just chock full of valuable information on essential oils. From listing properties of each oil, how to use the oils and brief description of where the oil comes from.

This app also has pictures showing where your vital points are on your hands and feet. These charts help greatly showing where on your hands and feet to put the essential oils to help alleviate pain for that area. For example, if you just mixed up a recipe to help heal a sciatica issue, the foot chart shows to put the essential oil mixture on the center of your heals.

It was enjoyable to write this book for you all. I would love to hear from you, if you would leave a review. It would be greatly appreciated.

10

Resources

Resources:

Reference Guide for Essential Oils- App on phone

Ward, R. [Fresh Start Nutrition]. (n.d.). *10 important essential oils to have on hand.* Fresh Start Nutrition. Retrieved December 8, 2024, from https://freshstartliveoak.com/about-us/

The 15 Best Essential Oils for Total Healing. (n.d.). Mudbrick Herb Cottage. Retrieved December 8, 2024, from https://www.herbcottage.com.au/blogs/aromatherapy/most-popular-essential-oils

Luebering, J. E. L. [Encyclopedia Britannica]. (2024, November 15). *https://www.britannica.com/topic/essential-oil.* Brittanica. Retrieved December 8, 2024, from https://www.britannica.com/topic/essential-oil

Kourkoutas, Y. (2017, November 5). *An Overview of the Biological Effects of Some Mediterranean Essential Oils on Human Health.* National Library of Medicine. Retrieved December 8, 2024, from https://pmc.ncbi.nlm.nih.gov/articles/PMC5694587/#:~:text=History%20of%20Pla

nt%20Essential%20Oils&text=Ancient%20Egyptians%20have%20use d%20aromatic,synthetically%20produced%20medications%20%5B3% 5D

Mendez, J. (2024, February 28). *The Intersection of Essential Oils and Modern Medicine.* Radha Beauty. Retrieved December 8, 2024, from https://www.radhabeauty.com/blogs/radha-blog/the-intersection-o f-essential-oils-and-modern-medicine?srsltid=AfmBOorXruMH0e1 9Z9O0NBMMMai_Va1WW3OE7bPzva7Dr2Dh_8gO3_Odt

Bohinen, S. (2023, September 5). *Top 20 Essential Oil Recipes.* Volantaroma.com. Retrieved December 8, 2024, from https://volantaroma.c om/blogs/recipes/top-20-essential-oil-recipes

New Direction Aromatics. (2017, June 21). *FRANKINCENSE OIL RECIPES TO ELEVATE YOUR WELL-BEING.* New Directions Aromatics. Retrieved December 8, 2024, from https://www.newdire ctionsaromatics.com/blog/frankincense-oil-recipes-to-elevate-your- well-being/#using-frankincense-oil-in-diffuser

Labaroma. (2021, September 15). *10 Essential Oil Recipes for Migraine.* Labaroma.com. Retrieved December 8, 2024, from https://www.labar oma.com/blog/10-essential-oil-recipes-for-migraine

Jenny. (2023, June 20). *Essential Oils for Eczema.* Essentialsholistic.com/. Retrieved December 8, 2024, from https://www.essentialsho listic.com/essential-oils-for-eczema/

Ecodrop. (2021, January 21). *4 Easy DIY Essential Oil Recipes for Anxiety Relief!* Ecodrop.co.uk. Retrieved December 8, 2024, from https://ecodrop.co.uk/blogs/beauty-products/essential-oil-recipes-f or-anxiety-relief

FERGUSON, J. (2020, August 3). *10 Diffuser Blends for the Cold and Flu Season!* inspiremenaturally.com. Retrieved December 8, 2024, from https://www.inspiremenaturally.com.au/blogs/news/10-diffuser-blen ds-cold-flu-season?srsltid=AfmBOorL1YqHeLkR5tWgxfPeXCGTKSu 29DGkPgmj1oMmluQKB8tcSgiW